The Better Bath vol. 3: Amazing Sugar Scrubs for Better Skin

Written by Lacey Jones

Disclaimer:

The information contained in this book is for general information purposes only.

While we endeavor to keep the information up to date and correct, we make no representations or warranties of any kind, express or implied, about the completeness, accuracy, reliability, suitability or availability with respect to the book or the information, products, services, or related graphics contained in the book for any purpose. Any reliance you place on such information is therefore strictly at your own risk.

None of the information in this this book is meant to be construed as medical advice. It has not been evaluated by the Food and Drug Administration.

Essential oils are powerful compounds. Consult with a medical professional prior to making changes that could impact your health.

Contents

Chapter 1: Introduction to the Better Bath Series of Books   6

Chapter 2: What Are Sugar Scrubs?   7

Chapter 3: Types of Sugar   9

Chapter 4: Types of Oil   11

Chapter 5: Essential Oils for Fragrance   13

Chapter 6: Making a Simple Sugar Scrub in 4 Easy Steps   15

Step 1: Choose the type of sugar you want to use.   15

Step 2: Choose a skin-safe oil and add it to the sugar.   15

Step 3: Add the Essential Oil   16

Step 4: Storing the Sugar Scrub   16

Chapter 7: The Basic Sugar Scrub   17

The Basic Sugar Scrub Recipe   18

Chapter 8: Lavender Sugar Scrub   19

Lavender Sugar Scrub Recipe   20

Vanilla Lavender   21

Lavender Lemon Sugar Scrub   22

Honey Lavender Scrub   23

Lavender Dry Skin Scrub   24

Sugar Chapter 9: Peppermint Scrub   25

Peppermint Sugar Scrub Recipe 26

Peppermint Tea Tree Sugar Scrub Recipe 27

Cucumber Mint Sugar Scrub Recipe 28

Peppermint Scrub Bars 29

Whipped Orange Mint Sugar Scrub 30

Chapter 10: Citrus Sugar Scrubs 32

Sweet Bergamot Sugar Scrub 33

Orange Blossom Scrub 35

Coconut Lime Body Scrub 37

Lemon Sugar Scrub 39

Chapter 11: Fruit Scrubs 40

Apple Pie Fruit Scrub Recipe 41

Applesauce Sugar Scrub 43

Banana Sugar Scrub 44

Cranberry Sugar Scrub 45

Pumpkin Spice Sugar Scrub 46

Peach Tea Sugar Scrub 47

Raspberry Lemon Sugar Scrub 48

Chapter 12: Coffee Sugar Scrubs 49

Coffee Sugar Scrub Recipe 50

Vanilla Cinnamon Coffee Sugar Scrub 51

Coffee Lavender Sugar Scrub 52

Chapter 13: Hot Cocoa Scrub 53

Hot Cocoa Scrub Recipe 54

Chapter 14: Green Tea Sugar Scrub   55

    Green Tea Sugar Scrub Recipe   56

Using a Sugar Scrub   57

Previous Books in the Series   60

Chapter 1: Introduction to the Better Bath Series of Books

This is the 3rd book in the Better Bath Series of books. The first book was on how to make bath bombs, which are little balls that fizz and release fragrances and oils when you toss them in the tub. In the second book, we covered fragranced bath salts that are easy to make and have a number of therapeutic benefits. This book is on sugar scrubs that can be rubbed into the skin to both moisturize and exfoliate it.

I wasn't sure what to expect when I started writing this series, but it's been well-received and I'm happy there are now a number of people who are using my recipes to improve their bath time experiences. All of the books in this series are available from Amazon.com and are available as both Kindle and paperback books. If you're new to the series and want to purchase the previous two books, there are links through which you can purchase them at the end of the book.

If you already own them, thanks for coming back. People like you are the reason I enjoy writing these books so much. I hope you enjoy this one as much as you've enjoyed the previous two!

Chapter 2: What Are Sugar Scrubs?

Is your skin in need of a little tender care?

If your skin is dry, cracked or suffering from the effect of time and age then sugar scrubs may be all that's required to return your skin to its former glory. Sugar scrubs will cost you a small fortune if you buy them at a boutique, which is surprising once you realize how simple and inexpensive they are to make at home. All you need is sugar, some sort of vegetable oil and maybe an ingredient or two to add fragrance to the scrub, and you're good to go.

A sugar scrub is a gentle scrub designed to exfoliate the skin. Over time, dead skin cells, oils, makeup, dirt and grime can build up on the surface of the skin and leave it looking dull and lifeless. *Exfoliation* is the process of removing the top layers of this build-up, revealing the healthy, soft skin beneath. When it comes to ingredients used to create exfoliating scrubs, sugar falls on the gentler end of the spectrum and is less abrasive than some of the other ingredients that can be used to make scrubs. I'd recommend starting with a sugar scrub first and then breaking out the bigger guns like salt and rice bran if the sugar scrub doesn't get the job done.

In addition to exfoliation, a good sugar scrub can carry a number of other benefits with them, including the following:

- **It moisturizes the skin.** Sugar scrubs have moisturizing properties, and the other oils and ingredients in the scrub can be tailored to hydrate the skin and add moisture to it.

- **It improves circulation.** The gentle massaging action used to rub the sugar into the skin improves circulation. Essential oils with rubifacient properties can be added to the scrub to further enhance circulation in the area to which the scrub is applied.
- **You may be able to reverse early signs of aging.** Sugar scrubs eliminate dead and damaged skin cells from the surface of the skin. Essential oils can be added that have tonic properties that will help tighten the skin and may eliminate or lessen minor wrinkles.
- **Improved skin health.** Skin blemishes like acne, blackheads, whiteheads and rashes become less likely when dead skin cells are removed from the picture. There is less of a chance of clogged pores and bacteria won't have a place to colonize and grow.

Sugar scrubs are a great way to pamper yourself at bath time. They can be used on your face, body, hands and feet and will leave your skin feeling great. You'll notice an almost instant change in the way your skin looks and feels, and you'll be left feeling like you wiped away years of damage.

Chapter 3: Types of Sugar

There are a number of varieties of sugar that can be used in sugar scrubs, with the key difference between the different varieties being the coarseness of the grains of sugar.

Generally speaking, you want to use the finer-grain sugars for facial scrubs, medium-grain sugars for your body and the larger grain sugars for the rougher parts of your body like your hands and the soles of your feet. The coarser the sugar, the more abrasive it's going to be. Larger granules of sugar will dig deeper into the skin, removing more skin cells when they're rubbed across it. The tradeoff is the larger grains can irritate sensitive areas and using too large a grain on sensitive skin can leave your skin feeling raw.

Here are the types of sugar you can use to make the recipes in this book:

- **White sugar.** This is your run of the mill white sugar. It's a fine grain sugar that's best when used in recipes that are going to be used on sensitive areas like your face.
- **Medium grain sugar.** Medium-sized sugar grains are a little bit coarser than white sugar, making them a good choice for scrubs that are going to be used on your neck, arms, legs and torso.
- **Brown sugar.** If you've got really sensitive skin, brown sugar might be your best option. It's softer than the other sugar types and is gentler.

- **Raw sugar.** This variety of sugar has larger grains that work well when used on tough areas of skin like your hands and the soles of your feet.

In addition to using the various types of sugar individually, they can be combined to create multi-purpose scrubs that can be used on the entire body. Be careful using the larger grains on soft, sensitive skin because they can cause irritation.

Chapter 4: Types of Oil

Rubbing dry sugar grains across your skin doesn't provide the same exfoliating properties as you get when you add some form of oil. Some people opt to use baby oil as the lubricating oil, but I prefer unrefined vegetable or nut oils because I'm not a big fan of mineral oils. You could get away with using baby oil if it's the only oil you have available, but the recipes in this book don't call for it.

The following oils are just a sampling of the many oils that are available that can be used in sugar scrub recipes:

- **Moringa oil.** This oil comes from the seeds of the *Moringa oilefera* tree. While most people haven't heard of Moringa oil, it's been in use for thousands of years. It's a light oil that spreads easily onto the skin and is found in a number of cosmetic and skin care products. It has anti-aging, antiseptic and anti-inflammatory properties and works well on dry, aging skin. The catch is this oil isn't cheap and it's often adulterated, so make sure you're buying your oil from a reputable source.
- **Tamanu oil.** This rare oil is sourced from Madagascar and is a soothing oil that offers relief from irritation, rashes, burns and sunburns. It's said to have regenerative properties and it's packed with antioxidants.
- **Jojoba oil.** While it's technically a wax, jojoba oil is a good oil to use when you have oily skin because it helps regulate sebum production. It

does leave behind a slightly waxy residue, so it's best to blend jojoba oil with other oils when you want to use it.

- **Rosehip oil.** If you're looking for a moisturizing oil, rosehip oil is one your better options. It's a highly-moisturizing oil with anti-aging properties.
- **Olive oil.** This oil is a middle-of-the-road oil that doesn't excel at any particular property, but is a decent oil that's readily available and is inexpensive.
- **Sweet almond oil.** This is one of my favorite oils for bath products. It's a moisturizing oil that's inexpensive and is gentle on the skin. Don't use sweet almond oil if you've got nut allergies.
- **Coconut oil.** Here's an oil that won't break the bank, but still manages to bring a number of beneficial properties to the table. Coconut oil is great at moisturizing the skin and will help heal dry and damaged skin. It can be used on most skin types and rarely causes an allergic reaction. Use coconut oils that are organic and unrefined for best results.

Generally speaking, if an oil is safe for use on your skin and has moisturizing properties, it will probably work well as an additive to sugar scrubs. Don't be afraid to experiment with different vegetable and nut oils until you find one you like.

Chapter 5: Essential Oils for Fragrance

If you've read any of my other books, you already know I prefer using essential oils for adding fragrance to my bath products. They're a better choice than synthetic fragrances because essential oils are all-natural and add a number of therapeutic properties to the products they're added to. Synthetic fragrances offer more variety, but they're made up of chemical compounds that don't bring anything other than a good smell to the table.

Essential oils are natural compounds that are the aromatic essence of plants. To put it simply, they're the reason plants smell the way they do. In addition to smelling great, essential oils contain a number of beneficial compounds that can do everything from moisturize the skin to improving circulation to helping you wind down and go to sleep. Essential oils can be combined to create oil blends that smell great and pack a potent punch.

There are a number of essential oils that are safe for most people to use. The essential oils used in the recipes in this book are used by a number of people to good effect, but don't assume they're perfectly safe for everyone.

Not all essential oils are safe for use, and oils that are safe for one person to use might not be safe for another. Some oils can cause skin irritation, some can interact with prescription medications by enhancing or dulling their effect and some might even cause uterine contractions in pregnant women. Because of the potential risk, it's important to consult with your physician to make sure the oils you're planning on using are safe for you to use. It's also important to test your essential oils by diluting them with coconut oil and applying them to a small area of your skin to see if there's a reaction. If there is, discontinue use immediately.

Chapter 6: Making a Simple Sugar Scrub in 4 Easy Steps

Making a simple sugar scrub is an easy process. In fact, it only takes 4 steps to make an effective sugar scrub that will do everything you need it to.

Here are the 4 steps required to make a sugar scrub:

Step 1: Choose the type of sugar you want to use.

This step's easy. You need to choose the sugar (or sugars) you want to use. Fine grain sugars are best for sensitive areas, and large grain sugars are best for areas with tougher skin. If you've got sensitive skin, go with brown sugar.

Step 2: Choose a skin-safe oil and add it to the sugar.

Decide on the type of oil you want to use. Most people opt for some kind of unrefined vegetable or nut oil. Organic oils will cost you more money, but are a better option because they won't contain trace amounts of the pesticides and other chemicals used to grow and treat plants that aren't grown organically.

If you're just starting out, I recommend extra-virgin coconut oil or sweet almond oil. There will be plenty of room for experimentation later. Add 1 part oil for every 2 parts of sugar you use. For example, if you've got 1 cup of sugar, you would add ½ cup of oil. If you're using 2 cups of sugar, you'd use a cup of oil.

Stir the oil and sugar together the best you can. The oil is going to settle to the bottom no matter what you do, so you'll have to give it a good stir the next time you want to use it.

Step 3: Add the Essential Oil

You can use one essential oil at a time or you can use oil blends, which are combinations of different essential oils. If you've got a favorite essential oil or oil blend, add it at this time. If not, I suggest starting with one of the milder oils like lavender essential oil. 5 to 20 drops of essential oil is all you're going to need for the recipes in this book.

Step 4: Storing the Sugar Scrub

The biggest concern with storing sugar scrubs is the oil that's used in the scrub might go rancid. You're going to want to store sugar scrubs in an airtight container and keep them away from heat, light and open air. Most sugar scrubs will last several months when stored at room temperature. It's best to make them in small batches, so you don't leave your sugar scrubs sitting out for long periods of time.

Chapter 7: The Basic Sugar Scrub

This recipe is the basic sugar scrub recipe from the previous chapter, but now it's in recipe form, so it's easier to follow. You'll be using this basic recipe to make the rest of the recipes in the book, so you might want to practice making it a time or two just to make sure you've got it dialed in.

I've used sweet almond oil in this recipe, but I could just have easily used extra-virgin coconut oil or any of a number of other oils that are good for the skin. Feel free to substitute it for your favorite oil.

The Basic Sugar Scrub Recipe

Ingredients:

2 cups sugar
1 cup sweet almond oil
5 to 10 drops of your favorite essential oil

Directions:

1. Combine the sugar and sweet almond oil and stir the two together.
2. Add the essential oil or oil blend and stir it in.
3. Store in an airtight container in a cool, dark place.

Chapter 8: Lavender Sugar Scrub

If you've been reading my books since the beginning, you've probably noticed a pattern with my first couple recipes in each book. I like to start with a basic recipe that can be used to make your own bath products with whatever essential oil or oil blend you'd like, and the next recipe is a recipe that calls for lavender essential oil.

This is done by design because lavender oil is a great essential oil to use as a jumping off point for those who are new to the world of essential oils. It's powerful in that it has strong healing and regenerative properties, yet is on the milder end of the spectrum when it comes to the potential for skin irritation, and most people can use lavender essential oil with no problems whatsoever.

Lavender Sugar Scrub Recipe

Ingredients:

2 cups sugar
1 cup sweet almond oil
10 to 15 drops of lavender essential oil

Directions:

1. Combine the sugar and sweet almond oil and stir the two together.
2. Add the lavender essential oil and stir it in.
3. Store in an airtight container in a cool, dark place.

Vanilla Lavender

The vanilla added to this recipe doesn't do much as far as therapeutic properties goes, but the fragrance melds with the lavender essential oil to create a fantastic fragrance that's tough to resist.

Ingredients:

1 cup brown sugar
1 cup granulated sugar
1 cup sweet almond oil
1 tablespoon vanilla extract
10 to 15 drops of lavender essential oil

Directions:

1. Combine the sugars and sweet almond oil and stir them together.
2. Add the vanilla and lavender essential oil and stir them in.
3. Store in an airtight container in a cool, dark place.

Lavender Lemon Sugar Scrub

We'll discuss lemon essential oil in the chapter on citrus sugar scrubs. For now, enjoy this lavender lemon sugar scrub.

Ingredients:

1 cup brown sugar
1 cup granulated sugar
1 cup sweet almond oil
10 to 15 drops of lavender essential oil
5 drops lemon essential oil

Directions:

1. Combine the sugars and sweet almond oil and stir them together.
2. Add the lemon and lavender essential oils and stir them in.
3. Store in an airtight container in a cool, dark place.

Honey Lavender Scrub

This recipe takes the basic lavender sugar scrub and adds honey to it. The honey is soothing to the skin and has antibacterial properties. It'll help knock down inflammation and is beneficial to most skin types.

Ingredients:

2 cups sugar
1 cup sweet almond oil
1 tablespoon raw honey
10 to 15 drops of lavender essential oil

Directions:

1. Combine the sugar, honey and sweet almond oil and stir them together.
2. Add the lavender essential oil and stir it in.
3. Store in an airtight container in a cool, dark place.

Lavender Dry Skin Scrub

This recipe features a double dose of ingredients that will moisturize and nourish dry skin. If you've got skin that's cracked and dry, this scrub might be able to help!

The Shea butter makes this recipe feel creamy and luxurious. It also helps the sugar slide across the skin, so it might be a good option for those with sensitive skin.

Ingredients:

2 cups sugar
½ cup sweet almond oil
½ cup Shea butter
3 tablespoons organic aloe vera gel
10 to 15 drops of lavender essential oil

Directions:

1. Combine the sugar, sweet almond oil, Shea butter and aloe gel and stir them together.
2. Add the lavender essential oil and stir it in.
3. Store in an airtight container in a cool, dark place.

Sugar Chapter 9: Peppermint Scrub

I absolutely love my peppermint sugar scrubs, but I've got to warn you. Peppermint essential oil is a powerful essential oil that will open up the capillaries in the area it's applied to and will get blood moving into that area. It produces a feeling similar to that of Icy Hot or Vicks Vapor Rub, and the way it feels may not be a pleasant experience for everyone. Keep it away from sensitive areas and be sure to test this sugar scrub on a small area of your body prior to wider application to make sure it's well-tolerated.

I like to give this sugar scrub as a gift around the holidays. Put it in a nice jar, attach a nice bow and a candy cane or peppermint or two, and you've got a great gift your friends and family will love. Don't forget to warn them about the strength of the peppermint oil!

Peppermint Sugar Scrub Recipe

Ingredients:

2 cups white sugar
1 cup coconut oil
5 to 10 drops of peppermint essential oil

Directions:

1. Combine the sugar and coconut oil and stir the two together.
2. Add the peppermint essential oil and stir it in.
3. Store in an airtight container in a cool, dark place.

Peppermint Tea Tree Sugar Scrub Recipe

How can you make the previous recipe even better? By adding tea tree oil to it, of course. Tea tree oil has a medicinal smell that not everyone is a fan of, but it's a great oil for skin care. Tea tree oil melds well with peppermint oil, creating a fragrance that is more pleasant than tea tree oil alone.

This sugar scrub is a great one to use if you have a cold. The fragrance should help clear out your stuffy head and will act as a decongestant.

Ingredients:

2 cups white sugar
1 cup coconut oil
5 to 10 drops of peppermint essential oil
5 drops tea tree essential oil.

Directions:

1. Combine the sugar and coconut oil and stir the two together.
2. Add the peppermint essential oil and tea tree oil and stir them in.
3. Store in an airtight container in a cool, dark place.

Cucumber Mint Sugar Scrub Recipe

This recipe adds the cooling and refreshing power of blended cucumbers to the previous recipe. If you don't have peppermint essential oil, you can crush a few tablespoons of mint leaves and add them to the recipe instead.

This sugar scrub won't last as long as some of the other scrubs because of the fresh cucumber used in it. Use it within a week of making it.

Ingredients:

2 cups sugar
1 cucumber
1 cup extra-virgin olive oil
5 to 10 drops peppermint essential oil

Directions:

1. Place the cucumber into a blender and blend until smooth.
2. Combine all of the ingredients and stir them together.
3. Store in an airtight container in a cool, dark place.

Peppermint Scrub Bars

Scrub bars are like sugar scrubs, but melt-and-pour soap is added to make it so the sugar scrub can be molded into bars that can be rubbed on your body. They're a great gift, and they work every bit as well as the sugar scrubs.

Ingredients:

2 cups white sugar
½ cup coconut oil
1 cup melt and pour soap
10 to 15 drops of peppermint essential oil

Directions:

1. Melt the melt-and-pour soap.
2. Stir the rest of the ingredients into it.
3. Pour the contents of the pot into silicon molds.
4. Leave the bars in the silicon molds until they've firmed up.
5. Pop the bars out of the molds.
6. Store in an airtight container in a cool, dark place.

Whipped Orange Mint Sugar Scrub

This sugar scrub is a little more work than the other scrubs in the book because it requires using a stand mixer with a paddle attachment to whip the sugar scrub until it turns creamy.

This recipe calls for Mandarin essential oil, which is a calming oil with a light, refreshing fragrance. It has healing properties and is a great oil to use on dry, cracked skin. Mandarin essential oil has the added benefit of repelling insects, so you might be able to use it to keep bugs at bay.

There's conflicting information out there regarding whether Mandarin essential oil is phototoxic. Mandarin leaf oil is strongly phototoxic, but regular mandarin oil isn't considered phototoxic and should be safe for most people to use.

Ingredients:

2 cups white sugar
2 cups coconut oil
10 drops of peppermint essential oil
10 drops of Mandarin essential oil

Directions:

1. Place the coconut oil in the fridge until it firms up.
2. Add the firm coconut oil and white sugar to the bowl of a stand mixer with a paddle attachment and blend on low until smooth.
3. Add the essential oils and blend them in.

4. Turn the speed up to Medium and blend for 45 seconds until the mixture starts to fluff up. It's done when it takes on a whipped texture.
5. Store the sugar scrub in an airtight container in a cool, dark place until you're ready to use it.

Chapter 10: Citrus Sugar Scrubs

There are a number of citrus essential oils available that can be used to create sugar scrubs. If you've ever bent an orange peel and watched the little geysers of liquid spray out of them, that liquid is essential oil. It's one of the easier oils for manufacturers to obtain and is inexpensive and readily available.

Citrus essential oils share some common attributes. They're great oils to use on oily skin, and they feature a refreshing citrus fragrance. One of the biggest benefits of citrus essential oils is their ability to tighten and tone the skin, which may help eliminate or lessen fine wrinkles.

Sweet Bergamot Sugar Scrub

This citrus sugar scrub calls for an essential oil from a fruit you probably haven't heard of unless you're familiar with the essential oils used in aromatherapy. Bergamot essential oil comes from the fruit of the Bergamot tree, a tree native to Southeastern Asia. The fruit looks like a cross between an orange and a grapefruit and turns a yellow color when ripe. The fruit generally isn't consumed, but the juice can be used as an ingredient in certain teas.

The fragrance of Bergamot essential oil is fruity with sweet citrus notes. It's a popular oil in perfumes and bath products because it has a floral quality to it that isn't found in the other citrus essential oils. Bergamot oil is a relaxing oil that's beneficial to those fighting a number of skin problems, including acne, psoriasis and even cold sores.

This recipe calls for brown sugar and is great for sensitive skin. As is the case with all of the recipes in the book, feel free to substitute other types of sugar as you see fit. I've used olive oil in this recipe because it doesn't have much fragrance and won't compete with the Bergamot oil. Feel free to use your favorite oil in place of the olive oil.

Bergamot oil is phototoxic and can cause a severe reaction when areas to which this oil has been applied are exposed to the sun within 24 hours of application. For this reason, Bergamot essential oil is best used on areas that won't be exposed to the sun when you head outdoors. Some suppliers sell bergaptene-free Bergamot oil that isn't phototoxic.

Ingredients:

2 cups brown sugar
1 cup extra-virgin olive oil
5 to 10 drops Bergamot essential oil

Directions:

1. Combine the brown sugar and olive oil and stir the two together.
2. Add the Bergamot essential oil and stir it in.
3. Store in an airtight container in a cool, dark place.

Orange Blossom Scrub

Orange blossom scrub uses neroli essential oil, which is also known as orange blossom oil. It smells more like a floral oil than it does a citrus oil because it's derived from the blossoms of the orange tree, but I've included it in this chapter because it's technically from a citrus plant. Neroli oil is one of the more expensive essential oils to buy because there isn't much essential oil found in orange blossoms and it takes a lot of flowers to make just a small amount of oil.

Neroli essential oil has a calming and soothing effect on the mind and body. Don't use this oil when you need to be focused and awake because it can be very relaxing. When used as part of a sugar scrub, it has rejuvenating properties that may help heal damaged skin and fade scars and stretch marks.

Unlike some citrus oils, neroli oil isn't phototoxic and can be used when you're going to be exposed to the sun.

Ingredients:

2 cups sugar
1 cup extra-virgin olive oil
10 to 15 drops Neroli essential oil

Directions:

1. Combine the sugar and olive oil and stir the two together.
2. Add the neroli essential oil and stir it in.

3. Store the sugar scrub in an airtight container in a cool, dark place.

Coconut Lime Body Scrub

If you don't like the way the fragrance of the coconut oil blends with the lime essential oil, you can swap the coconut oil out for an oil that doesn't smell like olive oil or sweet almond oil.

Lime essential oil smells just like the limes it's extracted from. It's a refreshing smell that will leave you feeling awake and alive. Lime essential oil is tonic by nature and can be used to help improve circulation, clear up acne, balance out oily skin and help with muscle aches and pains. It's also said to help clear up cellulite. Lime essential oil can be used to help heal scrapes, sunburns, insect bites and a variety of other skin conditions.

Lime essential oil can be phototoxic, so avoid exposure to the sun for at least 24 hours after it's been applied to the skin. If you are going to be exposed to the sun, only apply this scrub to areas that are going to be covered.

Ingredients:

1 cup white sugar
1 cup brown sugar
1 cup coconut oil
10 drops lime essential oil.

Directions:

1. Combine the sugars and coconut oil and stir the two together.
2. Add the lime essential oil and stir it in.

3. Store the sugar scrub in an airtight container in a cool, dark place.

Lemon Sugar Scrub

Lemon sugar scrub is another easy to make scrub that consists of only three ingredients. Lemon essential oil has similar properties to lime essential oil, including the phototoxicity. If you love the smell of lemon, you'll love this scrub.

Ingredients:

2 cups white sugar
1 cup sweet almond oil
5 to 10 drops lemon essential oil.

Directions:

1. Combine the sugar and sweet almond oil and stir the two together.
2. Add the lemon essential oil and stir it in.
3. Store the sugar scrub in an airtight container in a cool, dark place.

Chapter 11: Fruit Scrubs

When it comes to making scrubs that smell like your favorite fruits, you aren't going to be able to find essential oils for most fruits that aren't citrus fruits. What this means is you're going to have to look elsewhere to create fruit scrubs. There are synthetic fragrance oils that smell like pretty much every fruit you can imagine, but I prefer to use natural ingredients.

In order to keep your fruit scrub recipes natural, you're either going to have to find an essential oil or oil blend that smells similar to the fruit you want or you're going to have use the fruit itself (or the juice from the fruit) in your recipes. The problem with going the real fruit route is the scrubs won't last as long as they do when essential oils are used. I usually make them in small batches and try to use them within a week or two.

Apple Pie Fruit Scrub Recipe

Here's a recipe that smells like apple pie. When I first started making this recipe, I used to stir a couple tablespoons of apple juice into the recipe. Now I use Roman chamomile essential oil, which has a sweet fragrance that smells like apples, even though the oil is obtained from a completely different plant.

Roman chamomile oil is antibacterial, anti-inflammatory and antimicrobial by nature. It's a good choice for skin care products because of its healing properties. There is a chance of skin irritation, so test it on a small area prior to wider application.

When I'm making a small batch of this scrub, I'll often add a blended apple to it to make it smell even more like apple. If you add an apple to the recipe, peel it first, blend it in the blender and stir it into the sugar scrub in Step 1 in the recipe. Use scrubs that have real apple in them within a week of making them.

Ingredients:

2 cups sugar
1 cup coconut oil
10 drops Roman chamomile essential oil
1 teaspoon ground cinnamon or cinnamon extract

Directions:

1. Combine the sugar and coconut oil and stir the two together.

2. Add the Roman chamomile essential oil and stir it in.
3. Stir the cinnamon into the sugar scrub. If you're giving it as a gift, sprinkling a little bit of cinnamon on top will add aesthetic value.
4. Store the sugar scrub in an airtight container in a cool, dark place.

Applesauce Sugar Scrub

This recipe uses applesauce to make an apple-scented scrub. Unsweetened applesauce works great as an addition to a sugar scrub with one caveat. You've got to use this recipe quickly or store it in the fridge between uses. Even then, it's good for less than a week.

Ingredients:

1 cup white sugar
1 cup brown sugar
½ cup sweet almond oil
½ cup applesauce, unsweetened

Directions:

1. Combine the sugars, the applesauce and the sweet almond oil and stir them together.
2. Store the sugar scrub in an airtight container in a cool, dark place.

Banana Sugar Scrub

Use this recipe the day you make it for best results. It doesn't store well at all and will go bad quickly. I've cut down the amount of ingredients used in this recipe to account for the fact that it shouldn't be stored.

Ingredients:

½ cup white sugar
¼ cup coconut oil
½ ripe banana

Directions:

1. Combine the sugars and coconut oil and stir the two together.
2. Mash the banana and stir it into the coconut scrub until it's completely incorporated.
3. Use this recipe the same days it's made. It doesn't store well.

Cranberry Sugar Scrub

I'm not a huge fan of the fragrance of cranberries, but I made this recipe at the request of a friend and it actually turned out well. It's even better when you add 5 to 10 drops of Bergamot essential oil to it.

This recipe calls for fresh cranberries, so make it in small batches and use it quickly for best results.

Ingredients:

1 cup white sugar
1 cup brown sugar
20 to 30 whole cranberries
1 cup coconut oil
Optional: 5 to 10 drops Bergamot essential oil.

Directions:

1. Combine the sugars and coconut oil and stir the two together.
2. Blend the cranberries in the blender until smooth. Add them to the sugar scrub and stir them in.
3. Add the Bergamot essential oil at this time, if you plan on using it. Stir it into the scrub.
4. Store the sugar scrub in an airtight container in a cool, dark place.

Pumpkin Spice Sugar Scrub

This sugar scrub is interesting in that it doesn't contain anything remotely related to pumpkin, but still manages to smell similar to pumpkin pie. My husband thinks it smells more like gingerbread men, but either way it smells great.

Ingredients:

1 cup white sugar
1 cup brown sugar
1 cup coconut oil
1 teaspoon vanilla extract
½ teaspoon cinnamon
½ teaspoon nutmeg
½ teaspoon allspice

Directions:

1. Combine all of the ingredients and stir them together.
2. Store in an airtight container in a cool, dark place.

Peach Tea Sugar Scrub

It took me a while to figure out how to add a natural peach fragrance to my sugar scrubs. I tried blending peaches and adding them, but it really didn't smell like peaches and it turned slimy after a day or two.

I finally discovered that you can add peach fragrance to a sugar scrub by using peach tea. It works surprisingly well, and you get the added benefit of the antioxidants in the tea.

Ingredients:

2 cups brown sugar
1 cup coconut oil
4 peach tea bags

Directions:

1. Combine the brown sugar and coconut oil and stir the two together.
2. Open the tea bags and dump the contents of the bag into the sugar scrub. Stir it in.
3. Store the sugar scrub in an airtight container in a cool, dark place.

Raspberry Lemon Sugar Scrub

Be very careful when purchasing raspberry extract for this recipe. Some raspberry extracts aren't made with raspberries at all, and are instead made using other ingredients that are blended together to create a raspberry fragrance without actually using much by way of raspberries.

Some of these extracts are passed off as natural, but the natural ingredient they use comes from the anal glands of beavers. Sure, it's technically natural to the beaver it came from, but it isn't really something I want to rub into my skin.

Ingredients:

1 cup white sugar
1 cup brown sugar
1 cup coconut oil
1 to 2 tablespoons pure raspberry extract
5 to 10 drops lemon essential oil

Directions:

1. Combine all of the ingredients in a bowl and stir them together.
2. Store the sugar scrub in an airtight container in a cool, dark place.

Chapter 12: Coffee Sugar Scrubs

Sugar scrubs work well for most people, but they're only mildly abrasive and may not work to peel away thick layers of dry and dead skin. Ground coffee can be added to sugar scrubs when you need to call in the big guns.

The larger grains of coarsely-ground coffee will help exfoliate the skin, removing more dead skin cells than you'd remove with sugar alone. Additionally, the coffee contains antioxidants and other compounds that reduce inflammation and help eliminate skin problems. The caffeine in the coffee benefits your skin by toning and tightening it up, and it may be effective in reducing cellulite.

Coffee Sugar Scrub Recipe

Ingredients:

1 cup white sugar
1 cup coffee, ground
1 cup extra-virgin coconut oil

Directions:

1. Combine all of the ingredients and stir them together.
2. Store in an airtight container in a cool, dark place.

Vanilla Cinnamon Coffee Sugar Scrub

I really like the way this sugar scrub smells. The vanilla and cinnamon combine with the fragrance of the coffee to create an aroma that's tough to beat.

Ingredients:

1 cup white sugar
½ cup brown sugar
½ cup coffee, ground
1 cup coconut oil
1 teaspoon vanilla extract
½ teaspoon cinnamon

Directions:

1. Combine all of the ingredients and stir them together.
2. Store in an airtight container in a cool, dark place.

Coffee Lavender Sugar Scrub

There aren't too many ingredients that don't blend well with lavender. While coffee and lavender might not seem like a match made in heaven, they actually blend together to create a great-smelling sugar scrub.

Ingredients:

2 cups sugar
½ cup coffee, finely ground
½ cup dried lavender, crumbled
1 cup sweet almond oil
10 to 15 drops of lavender essential oil

Directions:

1. Combine the sugar, dried lavender and sweet almond oil and stir the two together.
2. Add the lavender essential oil and stir it in.
3. Stir the ground coffee in.
4. Store in an airtight container in a cool, dark place.

Chapter 13: Hot Cocoa Scrub

For the longest time, I thought relaxing in the tub while sipping a mug of hot cocoa was the number one most relaxing thing I could do. I truly believed this until I tried this sugar scrub. Now I believe using this sugar scrub and *then* hopping in the tub and sipping a mug of hot cocoa is number one. This recipes looks and smells delicious. If you love chocolate as much as I do, you're going to have to fight the urge to grab a spoon and dig in!

To top things off nicely, the cocoa in this recipe is good for your skin. It contains antioxidants and the caffeine in the chocolate will help tone and tighten things up a bit.

Hot Cocoa Scrub Recipe

Ingredients:

1 cup white sugar
1 cup brown sugar
1 cup coconut oil
3 tablespoon cocoa powder, unsweetened

Directions:

1. Combine the sugars and coconut oil and stir the two together.
2. Add most of the cocoa powder and stir it in. Sprinkle the remaining cocoa powder on top. If you're giving this scrub as a gift, you can include a few chocolate chips or chocolate shavings on top as well.
3. Store the sugar scrub in an airtight container in a cool, dark place.

Chapter 14: Green Tea Sugar Scrub

Green tea is one of my favorite teas to drink because it's good for your body and contains a number of antioxidant compounds. It's equally beneficial for your skin and is easy to make.

The first time I made this recipe, I used water instead of green tea and found the recipe to be a little lacking in the fragrance department. When I steeped the tea before adding it to the recipe, it created a much more aromatic sugar scrub.

Green Tea Sugar Scrub Recipe

Ingredients:

2 cups white sugar
½ cup sweet almond oil
1 cup water
4 green tea teabags (or 4 tablespoons green tea)

Directions:

1. Heat the water and place the tea bags into it and let it steep for 30 to 45 minutes.
2. Combine the sugar and sweet almond oil and stir the two together. Add 4 to 5 tablespoons of the steeped green tea to the mixture and stir it in. Discard the rest of the tea.
3. Cut 2 of the used tea bags open and stir the contents of the bags into the sugar scrub.
4. Store the sugar scrub in an airtight container in a cool, dark place.

Using a Sugar Scrub

Sugar scrubs are easy to use, but there are a few things you need to make sure you do in order to get the most from your homemade sugar scrubs. When used right, they'll gently exfoliate the skin while providing a number of therapeutic benefits. The exact benefits you'll reap depends on the rest of the ingredients used in the scrub.

Follow these directions to use your sugar scrubs:

1. **Open the sugar scrub and give it a good stir.** This step is important because when a sugar scrub is left to sit, the oils will sink to the bottom of the container, leaving the sugar at the top. Stirring the scrub combines everything, so you get the full power of the scrub.

2. **Scoop out a small amount of the scrub and massage it into the area you're trying to exfoliate.** I've found that small circles tend to work best, but you can experiment to see what works best for you. It's probably best to use just your hands on sensitive areas. You can use a loofah or a bath mitt to enhance the exfoliation in areas with tougher skin.

3. **Continue scooping the sugar scrub out and applying it to small areas until you've finished exfoliating the entire area you want to work on.**

4. **Leave the sugar scrub on for a few minutes and then rinse it off.** It's easiest to hop in the shower right after a sugar scrub.

When done right, a good sugar scrub will leave your skin feeling baby soft. Be aware that scrubbing too hard or for too long in sensitive areas can leave your skin feeling irritated and inflamed. If this happens, try going a little lighter on the scrubbing the next time around. You can also try switching the scrub to brown sugar or another fine grain sugar that isn't as abrasive.

Previous Books in the Series

If you're new to the Better Bath series and want the other two books, they're available from Amazon.com. The first book is about bath bombs and is available here:

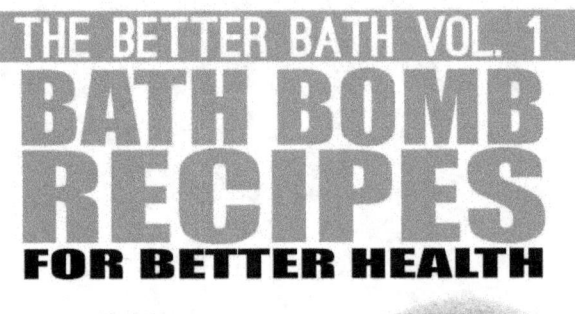
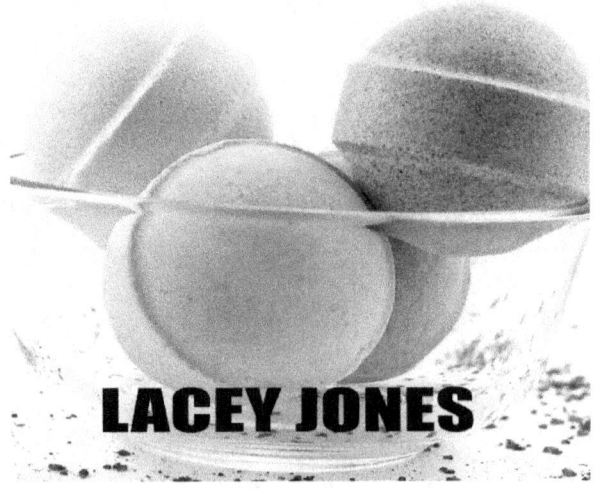

http://www.amazon.com/Bath-Bomb-Recipes-Better-Health-ebook/dp/B00RKJ2854/

The second book in the series teaches you how to make fragranced bath salts. You can purchase that book here:

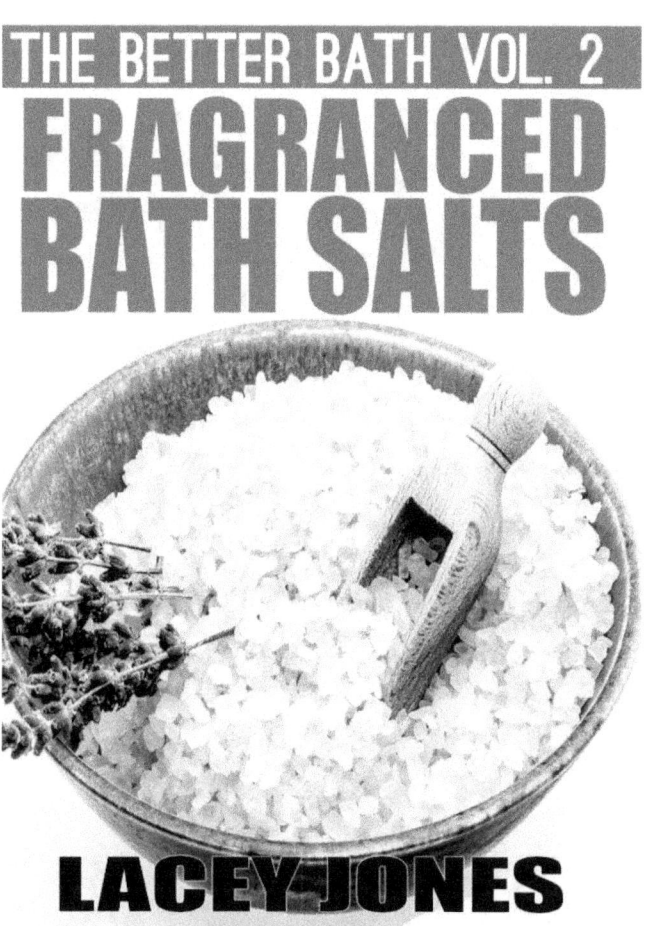

http://www.amazon.com/Better-Bath-vol-Fragranced-Salts-ebook/dp/B00ROX75Q8